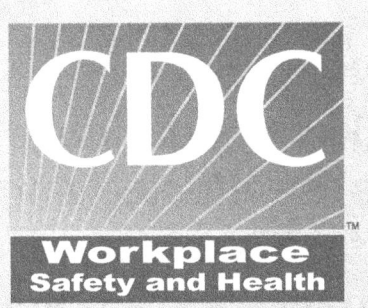

Evaluation of Respiratory Protection Practices for Employees at Federal Immigration and Customs Agency Workplaces – Nationwide

Marie A. de Perio, MD
R. Todd Niemeier, MS, CIH
Bradley S. King, MPH, CIH
Charles A. Mueller, MS

Health Hazard Evaluation Report
HETA 2009-0184-3126
April 2011

DEPARTMENT OF HEALTH AND HUMAN SERVICES
Centers for Disease Control and Prevention

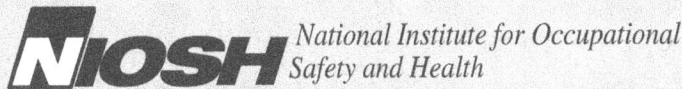

National Institute for Occupational Safety and Health

The employer shall post a copy of this report for a period of 30 calendar days at or near the workplace(s) of affected employees. The employer shall take steps to insure that the posted determinations are not altered, defaced, or covered by other material during such period. [37 FR 23640, November 7, 1972, as amended at 45 FR 2653, January 14, 1980].

CONTENTS

ABBREVIATIONS

μm	Micrometer
CDC	Centers for Disease Control and Prevention
CFR	Code of Federal Regulations
DO	Deportation officer
DHS	Department of Homeland Security
DRO	Detention and Removal Operations
FOD	Field office director
FOH	Federal Occupational Health
FPS	Federal Protective Service
HEPA	High efficiency particulate air
HHE	Health hazard evaluation
IEA	Immigration enforcement agent
NAICS	North American Industry Classification System
NIOSH	National Institute for Occupational Safety and Health
NIRU	National Incidence Response Unit
OI	Office of Investigations
OSHA	Occupational Safety and Health Administration
PAPR	Powered air-purifying respirator
pH1N1	2009 pandemic influenza A (H1N1)
PPD	Purified protein derivative
PPE	Personal protective equipment
RAC	Resident agent in charge
SA	Special agent
SAC	Special agent in charge
SCBA	Self-contained breathing apparatus
TST	Tuberculin skin test

The National Institute for Occupational Safety and Health (NIOSH) received a health hazard evaluation request from the American Federation of Government Employees in July 2009. The union was concerned about respiratory protection for employees of a federal immigration and customs agency.

What NIOSH Did

- We reviewed the agency's written respiratory protection procedures.

- We observed a respirator fit-testing session at agency headquarters.

- We surveyed employees across all agency workplaces about respiratory protection practices.

What NIOSH Found

- The agency's written respiratory protection procedures were comprehensive. However, written programs were reportedly not available at some agency workplaces.

- The quality of the respirator fit-testing procedures we observed was good. However, we did identify some areas that could be improved.

- Most employees who responded to the survey have face-to-face contact with immigrants in their current job. This contact puts them at risk of getting respiratory infections.

- Most employees who responded to the survey completed all required steps of the respirator fit-testing process. However, we did find some gaps between medical clearance and respirator training.

- Few employees reported being screened for tuberculosis in the last year.

What Managers Can Do

- Ensure that the written respiratory protection program is available at all agency workplaces.

- Follow all requirements in the OSHA Respiratory Protection standard.

- Require and arrange fit testing for employees at least annually.

- Develop and maintain clear written procedures for the use of respirators.

- Improve training provided to fit testers. Include more information on the technical capabilities of respirators and more specific instructions for the fit-testing procedure.

- Recommend tuberculosis screening for employees at least once a year.

- Recommend the influenza vaccine for employees every year.

What Employees Can Do

- Follow workplace procedures on use of respirators.
- Do a face seal check each time before you use a respirator.
- Get screened for tuberculosis at least once a year.
- Get the seasonal influenza vaccine every year.

Summary

NIOSH investigators assessed the respiratory protection program at federal immigration and customs agency workplaces nationwide. Overall the agency's respiratory protection program adequately protects employees from airborne infectious agents. However, several areas could be improved.

In July 2009, NIOSH received an HHE request from the American Federation of Government Employees. The union was concerned about respiratory protection for federal immigration and customs agency employees during the pH1N1 pandemic. NIOSH investigators reviewed the agency's written respiratory protection procedures, observed a respirator fit-testing session for employees at agency headquarters, and surveyed employees nationwide about respiratory protection practices.

We found that the agency's respiratory protection policy, the respirator medical evaluation questionnaire, the qualitative fit-testing protocol, and the slide presentation serving as training for fit testers were comprehensive. The quality of the observed respirator fit-testing procedures was good. However, we identified several areas that needed improvement.

Though the response rate for our survey was suboptimal with 2,218 responding employees, we found that that most respondents, particularly those from DRO and OI, have face-to-face contact with immigrants in their current job. This contact places them at risk for exposure to airborne infectious agents, including *Mycobacterium tuberculosis*, influenza virus, rubeola virus, and varicella zoster virus. Most respondents completed all of the steps required for respirator use (medical clearance, respirator training, respirator fit testing). However, some gaps between medical clearance and respirator training existed. We also found low employee compliance with respirator usage and annual tuberculosis screening. The written respiratory protection programs were not readily available in some workplaces.

The agency should maintain a written respiratory protection program for all workplaces to protect against airborne infectious agents and other respiratory hazards. The agency should require and arrange fit testing for employees at least annually and verify medical clearance prior to the fit test. Clear written procedures for the use of respirators should be developed and maintained, and specific indications for respirator usage should be included in training. Annual evaluations of the workplaces to ensure that the written respiratory protection program is being properly implemented should be conducted. Training provided to employees and fit testers should be improved to include more information on the technical capabilities of respirators and more specific instructions for performing face seal checks and for donning and doffing respirators. Employees who should undergo routine tuberculosis screening should be identified and informed. Finally, annual influenza vaccination should be recommended to all employees.

Keywords: NAICS 928120 (International Affairs), tuberculosis, TB, immigration facility, influenza, H1N1, measles, rubeola, chicken pox, varicella, infections, respirators, respiratory protection

On July 7, 2009, NIOSH received an HHE request from the American Federation of Government Employees. The request concerned the potential transmission of airborne infectious agents at federal immigration and customs agency workplaces nationwide. The union was concerned about respiratory protection provided to its employees during the pH1N1 pandemic. Though the initial focus of the request by the union was on DRO, employer representatives asked that we expand our evaluation to include all other divisions of the agency.

We discussed the request with union and employer representatives. We learned that the DHS issued interim guidance concerning PPE use by its employees in 2009 during the pH1N1 pandemic. Specifically, it provided guidance concerning voluntary use of an N95 respirator for employees in contact with persons known or suspected to have pH1N1 infection. It stated that managers and supervisors must provide their employees with a copy of Appendix D of the OSHA Respiratory Protection standard [29 CFR 1910.134].

While fit testing is not required for voluntary use of the N95 respirator, the agency launched a campaign, through NIRU, to qualitatively fit test more than 13,000 employees in July 2009 in anticipation of potential exposures to pH1N1 virus during the pandemic. This fit-testing campaign was completed in September 2009. All mission-essential personnel, defined by the agency, were required to be fit tested. Employees were required to complete an online respirator medical evaluation questionnaire through FOH. The total number of employees who underwent fit testing nationwide during this campaign was 13,777. The total number of employees successfully fitted for a respirator was not known at the national level.

Immigration and Customs Agency

The agency, part of DHS, is charged with protecting national security by enforcing the nation's immigration and customs laws. This agency employs approximately 19,000 persons in more than 400 offices nationwide and around the world. It is comprised of four main operational divisions: Office of Detention and Removal Operations, Office of Investigations, Office of Intelligence, and Office of International Affairs. Effective October 28, 2009, FPS, formerly an operational division of the agency, was placed under the National Protection and Programs Directorate of DHS.

DRO is the primary enforcement arm within the agency for the identification, apprehension, and removal of illegal, fugitive, and criminal immigrants from the United States. Approximately 7,600 employees work in DRO out of detention facilities, field offices and subfield offices, holding areas, and staging locations. OI is responsible for investigating, deterring, and interdicting threats arising from the movement of people and goods into and out of the United States. OI employs approximately 7,900 individuals. The Office of Intelligence collects, analyzes, and shares strategic and tactical data for use by the agency and the DHS management and operational units. The Office of Intelligence employs approximately 300 individuals. The Office of International Affairs employs approximately 300 individuals in more than 60 locations around the world. These international attaché offices coordinate investigations and law enforcement duties with international partners. The Office of State/Local Coordination, the National Firearms and Tactical Training Unit, the Office of Training and Development, and NIRU are also considered operational offices within the agency. NIRU develops, implements, and oversees key preparedness, prevention, response and recovery programs, and projects. It also supports and establishes uniformity of agency incident management and response efforts. The agency's management divisions employ more than 800 individuals, while the leadership offices within the Office of the Assistant Secretary employ more than 2,100 individuals.

Occupational medical clinical services, including immunizations, tuberculosis screening, and medical clearance for respirator use are provided to employees in partnership with the U.S. Public Health Service/FOH. Employees may be exposed to a variety of respiratory hazards while conducting law enforcement activities, emergency responses, or special operations.

Airborne Infectious Agents

Airborne transmission of infectious agents occurs by dissemination of either airborne droplet nuclei or small particles in the respirable size range ($\leq$ 10 µm) containing agents that remain infective over time and distance. These particles may remain suspended in air for long periods and may be widely dispersed by air currents. The microorganisms in these particles may be inhaled by susceptible individuals who have or have not had face-to-face contact with the infectious individual. Infectious agents that are transmitted by the airborne route include *Mycobacterium tuberculosis* [Riley et al. 1959; Haley et al. 1989; Beck-Sagué et al. 1992], rubeola virus (measles) [Bloch et al. 1985], and varicella zoster virus (chickenpox) [Leclair et al. 1980]. Although influenza viruses are thought to be mainly spread by droplet transmission (i.e., large respiratory droplets generated by coughing or sneezing and propelled over short distances), evidence for airborne transmission also exists [Bridges et al. 2003; Blachere et al. 2009; Lindsley et al. 2010a,b]. Detailed information on these airborne infectious agents can be found in Appendix A of this report.

A comprehensive program to prevent the spread of pathogens transmitted via the airborne route consists of engineering, administrative, and personal respiratory protection controls. Engineering controls such as the use of special air handling and ventilation systems are often used to help remove infectious agents in potentially high exposure areas such as isolation rooms or cells. Administrative controls include training employees on infectious control practices and medical surveillance programs for tuberculosis. In addition, respiratory protection is recommended for healthcare personnel and correctional and detention facility staff for protection against airborne infectious agents such as tuberculosis [CDC 2005, 2006]. More information on these controls can be found in Appendix A of this report.

Background on Respirators and Regulations

An estimated 5 million workers in 1.3 million U.S. workplaces are required to wear respirators at least some of the time while performing their job functions [OSHA 2010]. A respirator is a personal protective device that is worn on the face, covers at least the nose and mouth, and is designed to protect the wearer from inhaling hazardous airborne particles (including dust particles and infectious agents), gases, or vapors. Respirators should only be used as a "last line of defense" when engineering and administrative controls are not feasible or before these controls are implemented. Detailed information on respirators can be found in Appendix B of this report.

The current OSHA standard 29 CFR 1910.134, or Respiratory Protection standard, was implemented in April 1998 [29 CFR 1910.134]. It requires employers to provide respirators when they are necessary to protect the health of the employee. It also requires that employers develop and implement a written respiratory protection program when respirators are required. The standard contains requirements for program administration, worksite-specific procedures, respirator selection, employee training, fit testing, medical evaluation, respirator use, respirator cleaning, maintenance and repair, and other revisions. Employers must provide respirators, training, and medical evaluations at no cost to employees [29 CFR 1910.134]. The OSHA Respiratory Protection standard can be found at http://www.osha.gov/pls/oshaweb/owadisp.show_document?p_id=12716&p_table=standards.

ASSESSMENT

Our evaluation had three components: a review of the agency's written respiratory protection procedures, observation of a respirator fit-testing session at agency headquarters, and administration of an electronic survey about respiratory protection practices across all agency workplaces.

Review of Written Respiratory Protection Procedures

We reviewed the agency's respiratory protection policy, Directive Number 70005.1 dated January 31, 2007. FOH granted us access to the online respirator medical evaluation questionnaire for agency employees. We evaluated its components and compared it to the information mandated in Appendix C of the OSHA Respiratory Protection standard [29 CFR 1910.134]. We also reviewed the agency's qualitative fit testing protocol, including the fit-test checklist and instructions for fit testers. In addition, we reviewed the slide presentation that served as training given by FPS for fit testers.

Observation of a Respirator Fit-testing Session

A NIOSH investigator observed a qualitative respirator fit testing session at agency headquarters in August 2009. He observed a number of fit testers at various stations throughout the day and observed individual fit testers over successive fit tests. He listened to fit-tester instructions to employees being fit tested, noted specific procedures used for qualitatively fit testing the respirators, and gauged the level of understanding of the fit-testing procedure shown by both the fit tester and the employee being fit tested.

Electronic Survey

We surveyed employees about the implementation of respiratory protection and other infection control measures for airborne infectious agents at workplaces nationwide. Our objectives were to assess the completeness of employee coverage of the recently completed fit-testing campaign, identify barriers to undergoing and completing respirator fit testing, determine the success rates of respirator fit testing and reasons for unsuccessful tests, and assess adherence to other infection control measures for airborne infectious agents. We also looked at the role of the designated health and safety officer in the respiratory protection program and the respirator fit testers' attitudes towards the fit-testing process.

In January and February 2010, we disseminated an electronic survey to 19,424 current employees. The electronic questionnaire was sent to employees by agency managers through two broadcast e-mails. The survey was also placed on the agency intranet website. All employees were invited to participate. The questionnaire was anonymous and included no personal identifying information. Respondents had the option of returning the completed questionnaire directly to NIOSH investigators electronically or by fax. Surveys were collected over 6 weeks. The agency management and union sent multiple e-mail reminders to employees during the survey period. The survey included questions about work history, the recent respirator fit-testing campaign, tuberculosis screening, influenza vaccination, and workplace exposures to airborne infectious agents. Questions also addressed beliefs about and attitudes towards workplace practices and risk of acquiring infection, health and safety officers' knowledge about the respiratory protection program, and attitudes of fit testers towards the fit-testing process.

We summarized survey results using medians, ranges, and proportions as appropriate. Responses to questions about attitudes and beliefs were categorized as "expressed agreement" if respondents marked "agree" or "tend to agree," and as "expressed disagreement" if respondents marked "disagree" or "tend to disagree." Responses of "neither agree nor disagree" were left as is.

Review of the Written Respiratory Protection Procedures

The agency's respiratory protection policy, Directive Number 70005.1 dated January 31, 2007, provides guidelines for establishing and implementing a respiratory protection program. The policy states that the Health, Safety, and Environment Section within the Facilities Branch of the Office of Asset Management shall establish, implement, and maintain a respiratory protection program for employees. The program contains all of the basic elements required by OSHA including respirator selection, medical evaluation, respirator training, fit testing, respirator use, respirator cleaning, and maintenance and repair [29 CFR 1910.134]. It also clarifies the responsibilities within the program. While the Health, Safety, and Environment Section is responsible for overall coordination and implementation, NIRU is responsible for ensuring compliance with new or updated policies and guidance, specifically in the area of pandemic influenza. FPS is responsible for supporting the agency's programs in fit testing and training. However, it is uncertain if FPS maintains this responsibility because of organizational changes. Each program is responsible for ensuring that appropriate employees are identified, trained, and provided with PPE, and for developing standard operating procedures and/or guidance.

The agency's fit-testing procedures included all the elements required by the OSHA Respiratory Protection standard [29 CFR 1910.134] (Appendix B). The program requires medical clearance prior to fit testing. The online respirator medical evaluation questionnaire contains all questions found in the OSHA Respirator Medical Evaluation Questionnaire, Appendix C, to the OSHA Respiratory Protection standard [29 CFR 1910.134]. It also contains specific follow-up questions for "yes" answers to specific symptoms or problems. Upon completing the questionnaire, employees are immediately informed whether or not they have been medically cleared to wear a respirator. Employees are able to print a copy of the letter, and the system provides the clearance to the employee's Program Office and the Health, Safety, and Environmental Officer at headquarters. Employees who are not medically cleared by the questionnaire are sent for a follow-up medical evaluation.

The agency's fit-testing procedures incorporated respirator training during the fit-testing procedure; no separate training session existed for employees. The agency employed qualitative

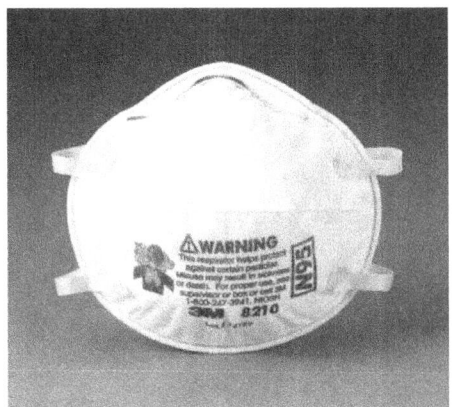

Figure 1. The 3M 8210 N95 respirator for which employees were fit tested. Photo © 2011 3M Company. All rights reserved.

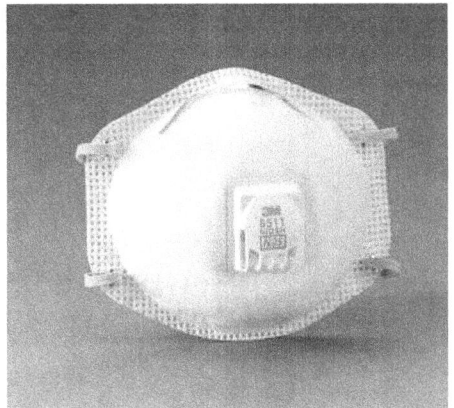

Figure 2. The 3M 8511 N95 respirator for which employees were fit tested. Photo © 2011 3M Company. All rights reserved.

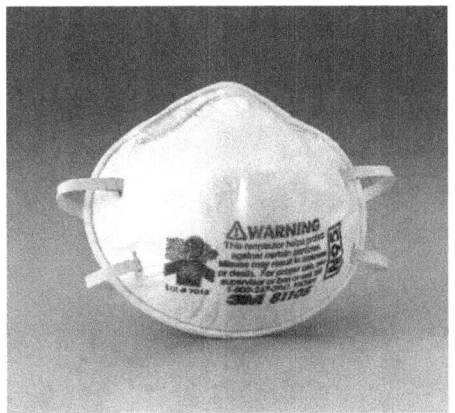

Figure 3. The 3M 8110S N95 respirator for which employees were fit tested. Photo © 2011 3M Company. All rights reserved.

fit testing consisting of a sensitivity test and a fit test. Fit testers were instructed about giving directions on proper donning and seal checking. The qualitative fit testing protocol contained the procedures for the sensitivity test and the fit test. Saccharin or Bitrex® was used as the challenge agent. Employees were required to perform eight simple tasks while wearing the respirator. The fit testing overview document stated that "if an individual detects the test solution at any time during the eight tasks, the N95 respirator will be refitted and retested. If the individual detects the taste a second time, he or she may be tested on another model of the N95 respirator. If an appropriate facial seal is not achieved with the second model, the individual cannot wear an N95 respirator and should be assigned to duties that would not expose him or her to airborne hazardous conditions." Fit testers were also given a checklist of instructions and actions for the fit-testing process. This checklist is comprehensive and contains the necessary details for each step of the process.

The slide presentation for training fit testers was thorough in the topics covered. It addressed the selection of respirators, general information on particulate filtering facepiece respirators, medical evaluation, and the details of administering a qualitative fit test. The training presentation also included the necessary equipment and materials, pretest preparations, and instructions for individuals being tested.

Observation of Respirator Fit-testing Session

On August 7, 2009, a NIOSH investigator observed the third of 3 days of qualitative respirator fit testing. Employees were fit tested for N95 filtering facepiece respirators in anticipation of potential exposures to pH1N1 virus during the pandemic.

Eleven fit-testing stations were set up, with each station's table approximately 8 feet from the next table. As employees arrived for testing after having been medically cleared to wear a respirator, they were checked in and directed to one of the fit-testing stations. Though the agency's fit testing overview document stated that employees would have two respirator model options during fit testing, three N95 respirators were available to employees on the observed testing date: 3M™8210, 3M8511, and 3M 8110S (Figures 1–3). The 3M 8210 and 8110S models are similar respirators and only vary in size.

The fit testers followed the qualitative fit-testing checklist developed by the agency for the saccharin sensitivity test and the respirator fit test. A 3M™ FT-10 fit-test apparatus was used for the qualitative fit tests. Bitrex® solution was available for employees who were not sensitive to saccharin. Depending on the agency program, the fit tester chose either the 3M 8210 model or the 3M 8511 model for fit testing. For example, OI employees were offered the 3M 8210 model; DRO employees were offered the 3M 8511. The reasoning behind this selection was practical; DRO agents were more likely to encounter pH1N1 exposures and to wear their respirators longer. The 3M 8511 model respirator has an exhalation valve that may make it more comfortable.

If the fit test failed, the employee was asked to wait 15 minutes, and the fit test was repeated using the same model respirator. If the fit test failed a second time, the smaller 3M 8110S model was tried. If the employee was successfully fit tested in one of the three respirator models, he or she was provided three respirators of that model to personally keep and store until needed.

Instructions Provided By the Fit Tester

The pertinent and required instructions provided by the fit testers were typically comprehensive and closely followed the agency's qualitative fit-testing checklist. Similar information was relayed to employees as they were being fit tested, irrespective of the particular fit tester. However, the NIOSH investigator noted a few deficiencies.

First, in a few instances, he observed that the top strap of the respirator was placed below the crown of the fit-test subject's head. The manufacturer's instructions state that the top strap is to be placed high on the top back of the subject's head, effectively crossing the crown of the individual's head [3M 2001]. While seemingly minor, incorrect placement of straps may result in a poor fit test.

Second, every fit tester observed required that the fit-test subject check for leakage around the face seal. However, the instructions on how to perform the face seal check did not often conform to instructions provided by the respirator manufacturer. For example, fit-test subjects were told to place the thumb and forefingers of both hands in C-shaped positions around the seal of the respirator and then inhale to identify any leaks. The fit testers did comment if they observed dimpling of the respirator, indicating a negative pressure was being achieved inside the respirator. However, these directions differ from the manufacturer instructions that state "To check the respirator-to-face seal, place both hands completely over the respirator and inhale sharply. Be careful not to disturb the position of the respirator. A negative pressure should be felt inside the respirator" [3M 2001].

Finally, in Part 1, Section A.6. of Appendix A of the OSHA Respiratory Protection standard, the OSHA-accepted Fit Test Protocol requirements, state "If the test subject is not familiar with using a particular respirator, the test subject shall be directed to don the mask several times and to adjust the straps each time to become adept at setting proper tension on the straps" [29 CFR 1910.134]. The NIOSH investigator observed that subjects were instructed to don the respirator a single time.

Qualitative Fit-testing Procedures

The fit-testing procedures generally followed Appendix A of the OSHA Respiratory Protection standard [29 CFR 1910.134]. However, in some instances, agency protocols differed from the OSHA-mandated procedures. First, the NIOSH investigator observed that some male agency employees with facial hair crossing the respirator sealing surface were fit tested and provided with the N95 respirators. Part 1, Section A 9 of the OSHA Respiratory Protection standard Appendix A, specifically states that "The test shall not be conducted if there is any hair growth between the skin and the facepiece sealing surface, such as stubble beard growth, beard, mustache, or sideburns which cross the respirator sealing surface" [29 CFR 1910.134].

Second, he observed that a selection of respirators was not available for each employee being tested. Due to logistical concerns, the model of respirator that the employee was fit tested on was preselected by the fit tester according to the division in which the employee worked. Part 1, Section A.1 of the OSHA Respiratory Protection standard states that "The test subject shall be allowed to pick the most acceptable respirator from a sufficient number of respirator models and sizes so that the respirator is acceptable to the user" [29 CFR 1910.134].

Finally, no mirror was available during the fit-testing procedures for the subjects to evaluate the positioning of the respirator on their face. Part 1, Section A.1 of Appendix A of the OSHA Respiratory Protection standard, states that "A mirror shall be available to assist the subject in evaluating the fit and positioning of the respirator" [29 CFR 1910.134].

Level of Understanding of the Fit-testing Procedure Shown by the Fit Tester

The NIOSH investigator learned that some fit testers did not have a solid understanding of the aerosols against which respirators are meant to protect the wearer. For example, many fit testers explained that an N95 respirator will filter 95% of particles down to 3 μm, which would include 100% of viruses, but may not be effective against smaller biological agents. In fact, N95 respirators are tested against and are at least 95% efficient in filtering particles with a 0.3 μm diameter, the size of particles that most easily passes through particulate filters. Although viruses and other particles may indeed be smaller, contrary to expectations, they do not penetrate the respirator filters as readily as particles with a 0.3 μm diameter, mainly because of capture mechanisms such as diffusion or electrostatic attraction. Therefore, the N95 respirator will effectively filter particles with diameters larger and smaller than 0.3 μm.

Cross-sectional Survey

We received 2,251 completed surveys by e-mail and by fax. Of this total, 33 respondents were excluded from our analysis because they reported working for FPS, which was no longer a program within the agency. Thus, we received 2,218 valid surveys out of 19,424 employees who were reported by management to have received the broadcast e-mail, a response rate of 11%. Of the 2,218 respondents, 1,648 (74%) were male, and 564 (26%) were female. The median age was 40 years, with a range of 21–74 years.

Work Characteristics

Employees from OI (49%) and DRO (45%) made up the majority of respondents. The largest number of respondents primarily worked in SAC or RAC offices (40%) and DRO field offices or suboffices (31%). Respondents working in all 50 states, the

District of Columbia, Puerto Rico, and Guam were represented. In addition, three employees working in Hong Kong, Italy, and Mexico responded. The most commonly reported job titles were SA or other investigations employee (37%), IEA (17%), administrative employee (17%), and DO (10%). The median number of hours worked a week was 50 (range: 16 to 110 hours). Other work characteristics of respondents are shown in Table 1. Seventy-six (3%) respondents reported being the local union representative at their workplace.

Of the 2,208 respondents who answered the question, 1,654 (75%) respondents reported having face-to-face contact with immigrants in their current job. Most employees in DRO (82%) and OI (74%) reported face-to-face contact with immigrants. Face-to-face contact was high among IEAs (99%), DOs (93%), DRO supervisors (87%), and SAs and other OI employees (83%), all job titles within DRO and OI. Respondents (n = 1,569) reported the median hours worked per week with face-to-face contact with immigrants was 6 hours (range: 0.15 to 60 hours).

Respirator Fit Testing Process Results

Respiratory protection characteristics of all respondents, DRO respondents, and OI respondents are shown in Table 2. Most (85%) respondents reported having undergone medical clearance to wear a respirator in the previous year. Of the 1,839 respondents who underwent medical clearance, most (98%) reported they were medically cleared.

Most (84%) respondents reported having had training on the proper use of respirators, and most (88%) reported having undergone respirator fit testing at their current workplace during the previous year. The most common reasons cited for not having respirator fit testing in the previous year were "I was not informed that fit testing was occurring," "I am a new hire," and "I don't know." Of the respondents who reported having face-to-face contact with immigrants, 88% reported undergoing medical clearance, 87% reported undergoing respirator training, and 92% reported undergoing respirator fit testing.

Table 1. Work characteristics of survey respondents

Work Characteristic	No. Respondents (%) n = 2,031–2,213*
Agency program	
OI	1,078 (49)
DRO	996 (45)
Office of the Principal Legal Advisor	59 (3)
Office of Intelligence	40 (2)
Other	40 (2)
Type of primary workplace	
SAC, deputy SAC, assistant SAC, RAC office	892 (40)
DRO field office or suboffice	687 (31)
Other federal government building	259 (12)
Service processing center	111 (5)
Contract detention facility	90 (4)
Staging facility	23 (1)
Other	143 (6)
Location of primary workplace	
South region†	615 (30)
West region‡	573 (28)
Northeast region§	505 (25)
Midwest region¶	338 (17)
Job title	
SA, other investigations employee	810 (37)
IEA	383 (17)
Administrative employee	368 (17)
DO	210 (10)
DRO supervisor	179 (8)
Investigations supervisor	138 (6)
Attorney	59 (3)
Intelligence officer, specialist, supervisor, director	29 (1)
Other	35 (2)

*Samples sizes ranged 2,031–2,213 due to missing values.
†South region includes District of Columbia, Virginia, North Carolina, South Carolina, Georgia, Florida, Tennessee, Alabama, Mississippi, Arkansas, Louisiana, Texas, Oklahoma, New Mexico, and Puerto Rico.
‡West region includes Colorado, Wyoming, Montana, Idaho, Utah, Nevada, Washington, Oregon, California, Arizona, Hawaii, Alaska, and Guam.
§Northeast region includes Maine, New Hampshire, Vermont, Massachusetts, Rhode Island, Connecticut, New York, New Jersey, Pennsylvania, West Virginia, Maryland, and Delaware.
¶Midwest region includes Michigan, Ohio, Wisconsin, Illinois, Indiana, Kentucky, Missouri, Nebraska, Minnesota, Iowa, North Dakota, South Dakota, and Kansas.

Most (97%) of the 1,943 respondents who underwent fit testing and reported whether or not they were successfully fitted for a respirator reported they were successfully fitted. The most common reasons cited for not being successfully fitted were "I could not get a tight seal of the respirator on my face," "the correct size respirator for my face was not available," "I have facial hair," and "I could not smell/taste the test aerosol used for fit testing."

Most (75%) of the 2,161 respondents who answered all questions related to the respirator fit-testing process reported completing all steps of the process (i.e., medical clearance, respirator training, and fit testing) and were successfully fitted for a respirator. Of the 2,161 respondents, 30 (1%) completed all steps but were not successfully fitted for a respirator. A total of 189 (9%) respondents reported completing none of the three steps of the respirator fit testing process while 313 (14%) respondents reported not completing one or two steps of the process.

Respirator Access and Usage

A total of 1,968 (89%) respondents reported having access to an N95 filtering facepiece respirator at their current workplace, with 96% of DRO respondents and 89% of OI respondents reporting access. Of those who reported having face-to-face contact with immigrants, 92% reported having access to an N95 respirator.

Regarding respirator usage, 235 (11%) respondents reported ever wearing an N95 filtering facepiece respirator, and 25 (1%) respondents reported wearing another type of respirator (type unspecified) at their current workplace in the previous year. Of those respondents who reported wearing an N95 filtering facepiece respirator, 79 (34%) reported wearing it for contact with someone with tuberculosis, while 144 (61%) reported wearing it for contact with someone with pH1N1or other influenza-like illness. Other reasons not listed in the survey but written in by respondents included for precautionary use (n = 8) and contact with narcotics (n = 7). Of those respondents who reported wearing another type of respirator, 5 (20%) reported wearing it for contact with someone with tuberculosis, while 2 (8%) reported wearing it for contact with someone with pH1N1 or other influenza-like illness. Other reasons not listed in the survey but written in by respondents included for training (n = 5) and hazardous material exposure (n = 6).

Table 2. Respiratory protection characteristics of survey respondents

Practice	Number Total Respondents (%)	Number DRO Respondents (%)	Number OI Respondents (%)
Underwent medical clearance to wear respirator	1,878 of 2,211 (85)	883 of 994 (89)	948 of 1,075 (88)
Cleared to wear respirator*	1,802 of 1,839 (98)	855 of 867 (99)	905 of 926 (98)
Had respirator training	1,852 of 2,209 (84)	898 of 993 (90)	912 of 1,074 (85)
Underwent respirator fit testing	1,955 of 2,216 (88)	949 of 996 (95)	964 of 1,077 (90)
Successfully fitted†	1,885 of 1,943 (97)	925 of 945 (98)	925 0f 957 (97)

*The denominators include those respondents who underwent medical clearance.
†The denominators include those respondents who underwent respirator fit testing.

When broken down by agency program, 176 (18%) of 994 DRO respondents reported ever wearing an N95 filtering facepiece respirator, and 14 (1%) of 991 DRO respondents reported wearing another type of respirator at their current workplace in the previous year. Fifty-five (5%) of 1,078 OI respondents reported wearing an N95 filtering facepiece respirator, and 11 (1%) of 1,076 OI respondents reported ever wearing another type of respirator at their current workplace in the previous year. Job titles with the highest percentages of respondents reporting ever wearing an N95 respirator in the previous year were IEA (26%), DO (16%), and DRO supervisor (16%).

Of the 235 respondents who reported ever wearing an N95 filtering facepiece respirator at their current workplace in the previous year, 214 (91%) had undergone respirator training during the previous year. In addition, 225 (96%) reported undergoing respirator fit testing in the previous year. Of the 223 respondents who reported ever wearing an N95 respirator and undergoing a respirator fit test in the previous year and reported whether or not it was successful, 218 (98%) reported having a successful fit test.

Most (69%) respondents expressed agreement that their workplace does its best to have respirators available when they are needed, and most (62%) respondents expressed agreement that the appropriate respirator is always available for them when they need it. A smaller percentage of respondents (46%) expressed agreement that their workplace has clear written procedures for the use of respirators.

Infectious Diseases Exposures and Infection Control Practices

Most (59%) respondents expressed agreement that their workplace does its best to protect workers from exposure to respiratory infections. Although most (62%) respondents expressed agreement that they were at risk of catching influenza, tuberculosis, or other respiratory infection due to their job, fewer (33%) respondents expressed agreement that they frequently worry about catching influenza, tuberculosis, or other respiratory infection due to their job.

The numbers of respondents who reported having face-to-face contact with persons with known infections in the previous year were 403 (18%) for tuberculosis, 28 (1%) for measles, and 96 (4%) for chicken pox. The number of respondents who reported having face-to-face contact with persons with known pH1N1 between April 2009 and survey administration was 376 (17%). Of the 403 respondents who reported having face-to-face contact with persons with known tuberculosis, 68 (17%) of them reported wearing an N95 respirator during contact.

Regarding tuberculosis screening practices, 466 (21%) respondents reported having had a tuberculosis skin test or PPD test in the previous year. The most common places where respondents received their last tuberculosis skin test were an FOH clinic (50%) and a personal physician's office (27%). Twenty (4%) respondents reported receiving their last tuberculosis skin test at their workplace. The most common reasons cited by respondents who did not have a tuberculosis skin test in the previous year for not having one were, "I did not think I needed a tuberculosis skin test" (48%), "I have not been told that I need to get tested" (46%), "I have not felt sick" (21%), and "I do not know where to get tested" (12%). (Respondents could cite more than one reason.) Six percent of respondents reported previously testing positive or having a history of latent or active tuberculosis.

A total of 273 (28%) DRO respondents and 178 (16%) OI respondents reported having had a tuberculosis skin test in the previous year. Of the total respondents who reported having face-to-face contact with immigrants, 378 (23%) reported having had a tuberculosis skin test in the previous year. Job titles with the highest percentage of respondents reporting having had a tuberculosis skin test in the previous year were IEA (38%), DRO supervisor (26%), administrative personnel (18%), special agent or other OI employee (18%), and DO (17%). Of the 35 respondents from the "other" category for job title, 34% reported having had a tuberculosis skin test in the previous year.

A total of 997 (45%) respondents reported having received the seasonal influenza vaccine between October 1, 2008, and March 31, 2009. The most common places where respondents received this seasonal influenza vaccine were at an FOH clinic (37%), at their personal physician's office (34%), and at a pharmacy or store (8%). Fifty-four (5%) respondents reported receiving their seasonal influenza vaccine at their workplace. The most common reasons cited by the 1,215 respondents who did not have a seasonal influenza vaccine during the above period were "I didn't think I needed the flu vaccine" (42%), "I did not think the influenza vaccine would keep me from getting the flu" (23%), "other" reason (15%), "It was inconvenient for me to get vaccinated" (11%), "The influenza vaccine causes the flu or makes me sick" (10%), and "the influenza vaccine is not safe (8%). (Respondents could cite more than one reason.) "Other" reasons included "I did not want it" and "I never get it."

Designated Safety Officer

Of the 111 designated safety officers throughout the agency, 70 completed the survey for a response rate of 63%. They represented 3% of the total survey respondents. Of these 70 safety officers, 33 (47%) were from OI, 32 (46%) were from DRO, 4 (6%) were from the Office of Intelligence, and 1 (1%) was from the Office of the Principal Legal Advisor. Of the 69 respondents who answered the subsequent questions, 30 (43%) reported having a written respiratory protection program at their workplace, 17 (25%) reported not having one, and 22 (32%) reported not knowing. Sixteen (50%) DRO safety officers and 18 (56%) OI safety officers reported either not having a written respiratory protection program or not knowing they had one. Excluding those respondents who worked in "other" workplaces not listed in the survey, the two most common workplaces of the safety officers that reported either not having a written respiratory protection program or not knowing whether they had one were SAC or RAC office (n = 13) and DRO field office or suboffice (n = 12). These two workplaces are the most common workplaces in the agency.

Most of the 30 responding safety officers who reported having a written respiratory protection program reported that their written program addressed all of the areas listed in the OSHA Respiratory Protection standard [29 CFR 1910.134]. Between 90% and 97% of responding safety officers reported that their workplace's written respiratory protection program addressed most of the individual areas listed in the standard. However, fewer reported that their workplace's program addressed medical evaluations of employees for respirator use (83%); cleaning, disinfecting, storing, inspecting, repairing, and discarding respirators (73%); and evaluating the effectiveness of the program (70%).

Of the 69 designated safety officers, 23 (33%) reported they were the respiratory protection program administrator at their workplace. Nine of these 23 safety officers reported overseeing these programs without having received specific respirator training. Of the 13 who did receive training, the most common sources of training reported were on-the-job training (n = 6), a multi-day respirator use training course (n = 5), and a one-day respirator use training course (n = 3).

Seven (10%) of the 69 designated safety officers reported they were involved in the selection of respirators for employees at their workplace. Of 69 safety officers, 68 reported that some type of mask or respiratory protection was available at their workplace. These safety officers reported availability of surgical masks (29%), dust masks (26%), N95 filtering respirators (96%), and full facepiece elastomeric air purifying respirators (3%). Half-mask elastomeric air purifying respirators and PAPRs were not reported to be available at their workplace. One safety officer answered "I don't know" to the question about what type of respiratory protection was available at his or her workplace.

Fit Testers

A total of 245 (11%) of 2,160 respondents reported having been trained to become a respirator fit tester, 150 in the previous year and 95 more than 1 year earlier. The agency reported that 319 employees were trained as fit testers during the fit-testing campaign of 2009, giving a response rate of 47% among fit testers. The median number of employees fit tested by the 119 responding fit testers from May 2009 to survey administration was 20 employees (range: 0–400 employees).

Twenty-three fit testers who trained in the previous year and 91 fit testers who trained more than 1 year earlier did not answer the subsequent question of who trained them. Of the 131 fit testers who did answer subsequent questions, most (74%) reported being trained by another agency employee, while 24 (18%) reported being trained by FPS HazMat Technicians fit testers.

In addition, between 94 and 106 fit testers did not answer subsequent questions regarding their comfort level with their expertise. Of those who did answer these questions, 109 (72%) expressed agreement that they feel comfortable conducting a qualitative respirator fit test on an employee, 105 (72%) expressed agreement that they feel comfortable giving instructions to fit-test subjects during the fit-testing session, and 79 (54%) expressed agreement that they feel comfortable answering technical questions about respirator effectiveness. Ninety-seven (70%) fit testers expressed agreement that the fit tests that they conduct are accurate, while 87 (62%) fit testers expressed agreement that the training session they attended adequately prepared them to conduct fit tests.

DISCUSSION

While the response rate to our survey was suboptimal, our results yield useful information regarding employee exposures to airborne infectious agents and respiratory protection at the agency. Most (75%) employees who responded to the survey, particularly those from DRO and OI, reported having face-to-face contact with immigrants in their current job, which places them at risk for exposure to airborne infectious agents. Almost two thirds of respondents believe they are at risk of acquiring a respiratory infection due to their job, and almost one third responded that they frequently worry about this risk. In addition, the percentages of respondents who reported having face-to-face contact with persons with known infections were 18% for tuberculosis in the previous year and 17% for pH1N1 between April 2009 and the survey administration. This level of contact indicates that a comprehensive program to protect employees from airborne infectious diseases hazards is appropriate. The respirator fit-testing process appears to be comprehensive, as most (75%) responding employees completed all of the required steps of the respirator fit-testing process and were successfully fitted. However, some gaps existed particularly in the areas of medical clearance and respirator training. Our findings suggest that verifying documentation of medical clearance did not always occur prior to fit testing. In addition, our findings indicate that the training that was supposed to have been included in the fit-testing session occasionally either did not occur or was suboptimal.

The rate of medical clearance to wear a respirator for those undergoing evaluation was high at 98%. The online respirator medical evaluation questionnaire administered through FOH is comprehensive and contains all of the questions found in the OSHA Respirator Medical Evaluation Questionnaire, Appendix C, to the OSHA Respiratory Protection standard [29 CFR 1910.134]. This questionnaire is used for medical evaluation and to identify persons who require additional examination. A study of Department of Energy workers found that a similar medical evaluation questionnaire demonstrated a sensitivity of 100% for the detection of workers requiring work restrictions [Pappas et al. 1999]. This study supports the use of a self-administered questionnaire for medical clearance in certain settings such as a large federal agency.

The rate of a successful fit test for those undergoing fit testing was high at 97%. The most common reasons cited by respondents for not being successfully fitted for a respirator were "I could not get a tight seal of the respirator on my face" and "the correct size respirator for my face was not available." These reasons suggest that a larger selection of N95 respirators than the three 3M models might need to be available. The next most common reason cited by respondents for not being successfully fitted was "I have facial hair." This finding, coupled with our observation that some employees with facial hair between the face and the respirator sealing surface were being fit tested, suggests that fit testers need to improve compliance with the OSHA Respiratory Protection standard [29 CFR 1910.134] and deny a fit test to those employees with facial hair.

The agency's tuberculosis exposure control plan states that "all employees with potential exposure to detainees or others with active tuberculosis will be provided N95 facemasks or HEPA respirators. Employees must wear the facemasks in high hazard settings where administrative and engineering controls are not likely to provide adequate protection. High hazard settings include close contact with a suspected active case of tuberculosis and entering a tuberculosis isolation room when it is occupied by an individual with a known or suspected active case of tuberculosis."

The term "facemask" should be replaced with "respirator" in this plan to prevent confusion with surgical face masks, which are not appropriate protection from exposure to tuberculosis. Furthermore, the term "HEPA respirator" is an outdated term and should also be avoided. Instead, the level of protection and the level of filtration should be noted (e.g., PAPR with high-efficiency filters).

Though most respondents reported having access to N95 filtering facepiece respirators, respirator usage by respondents for contact with persons with known tuberculosis was low at 17%. This indicates that employee training should emphasize the indications for respirator use, which include close contact with persons with active tuberculosis.

We found low compliance with tuberculosis screening agencywide. The agency's tuberculosis exposure control plan states that all employees "who are at risk for exposure to tuberculosis" are included in the tuberculosis surveillance and screening program. Clarification on how a determination of an employee's risk for exposure to tuberculosis is made is necessary. The plan requires baseline PPD testing during all preplacement examinations. The employee can provide written documentation of the results of a test performed within 6 months of the date of preplacement testing. The plan states that "baseline testing will be followed, at least annually, by PPD testing and risk assessment." However, almost half of responding employees were not aware of the recommendation that they undergo at least annual tuberculosis screening.

Use of respirators or facemasks was not recommended by CDC for workers in nonhealthcare occupational settings for general work activities during the pH1N1 pandemic [CDC 2009]. CDC's "Prevention Strategies for Seasonal Influenza in Healthcare Settings" currently recommends use of facemasks (not N95 respirators) by workers for most forms of contact with persons with confirmed or suspected influenza in healthcare settings [CDC 2010b]. In addition, CDC's "Interim Guidance for the Use of Masks to Control Influenza Transmission" does not currently recommend the use of facemasks or respirators for individuals in community settings who are not ill [CDC 2010a].

Less than half of the responding safety officers reported having a written respiratory protection program at their workplace, despite the availability of an agencywide written program. It is possible that a written respiratory protection program may actually have been in existence at their workplace and the safety officer may not have known this. Nevertheless, safety officers should be knowledgeable about this program. These results are comparable to a survey conducted by the Bureau of Labor Statistics, U.S. Department of Labor, which found that only 35% of private industry workplaces that required respirator use had established a written respiratory protection program adopted by management [BLS and NIOSH 2003].

Most responding safety officers reported having a written respiratory protection program and reported it had all of the required components of the OSHA Respiratory Protection standard [29 CFR 1910.134]. Only one third of safety officers reported they were the respiratory protection program administrator at their workplace, and fewer reported they were involved in the selection of appropriate respirators for employees at their workplace. These findings demonstrate that the role of safety officers in the respiratory protection program should be clarified and strengthened.

Most (72%) fit testers felt comfortable conducting a qualitative respirator fit test and giving instructions to fit-test subjects during the fit-testing session. Nevertheless, we observed that improvements can be made when giving instructions on proper donning of the respirator and conducting a seal check. Also, fewer (62%) fit testers thought that the training session adequately prepared them to conduct fit testing and fewer (54%) felt comfortable answering technical questions about respirators. These findings are consistent with our observation that some fit testers did not appear to have a solid understanding of the filtering efficiency of respirators during the fit-testing session. Though the slide presentation that served as training for fit testers given by FPS was thorough, more details on filtering efficiency and the technical capabilities of respirators could be added.

Our evaluation was subject to some limitations. We observed only 1 day of fit testing; thus, these observations may not be representative of all fit-testing sessions and all fit testers across the agency. Also, while we reviewed the slide presentation that served as training for fit testers, we did not observe an actual training session. The response rate to our survey was 11% despite two e-mail reminders from employer and union representatives. We believe several factors may have contributed to the low response rate. First, at the Office of the Chief Information Officers' directive, we did not have direct contact with all employees and rather relied on this office to disseminate the invitation and survey for us. Employees may have been uncomfortable responding to a survey sent out by management despite being told it was confidential. Second, although we intended to invite all agency employees to participate in the survey, the e-mail invitation specifically encouraged participation among employees who had participated in the recent respirator fit-testing program. Third, though employees were instructed not to reply to the e-mail from the agency's broadcast and to send their completed surveys to our dedicated e-mail address, it is possible we did not receive all completed surveys due to incorrect return. Fourth, the agency disseminated our survey on January 14, 2010, 2 days after the earthquake in Haiti. Employees from many agency programs were involved in this response. Finally, we were unable to verify the number of employees who actually received this e-mail, so our response rate may be an underestimation.

The response rate to our survey is lower than those seen in other electronic surveys (mean response rates between 19% and 40%), but lower rates are seen in larger surveys, workplace surveys, and surveys not offering incentives [Jones and Pitt 1999; Cook et al. 2000; Sheehan 2001; Manfreda and Vehovar 2002; Kaplowitz et al. 2004; Shih and Fan 2008]. Nevertheless, our relatively low response rate raises the possibility that our results are not representative of all agency employees, especially employees from the management and leadership offices. An additional limitation of this evaluation was that the survey administration period was in January and February 2010. Because the respirator fit-testing campaign ended in September 2009, this may have limited respondents' ability to recall certain information about the process and may have affected our results.

CONCLUSIONS

Most responding agency employees, particularly those from DRO and OI, reported having face-to-face contact with immigrants in their current job, which places them at risk for potential exposure to airborne infectious agents. The quality of the observed respirator fit-testing procedures was good, and most responding employees completed all of the required steps of the respirator fit testing process. However, some gaps with respect to medical clearance and respirator training existed. We also found that written respiratory protection programs were lacking in some workplaces and that employee compliance with respirator usage and that annual tuberculosis screening was low.

RECOMMENDATIONS

A comprehensive infection control program, with attention to airborne infectious agents, is necessary at agency workplaces where employees have the potential for contact with immigrants. The program should include all of the following: education of employees, hand hygiene, respiratory hygiene and cough etiquette, procédures for the screening and management of immigrants with fever and respiratory symptoms, exclusion of ill employees from work, influenza vaccination, annual tuberculosis screening of employees, and a written respiratory protection program for employees. Although respirator use was the focus of our evaluation, use of respirators and other PPE ranks lowest in the hierarchy of controls and is a last line of defense for employees against hazards that cannot otherwise be eliminated or controlled. Careful attention to elimination of potential exposures, engineering controls, and administrative controls will reduce the need to rely on PPE, including respirators.

On the basis of our findings, we recommend the actions listed below to create a more healthful workplace. We encourage the agency to use a labor-management health and safety committee or working group to discuss the recommendations in this report and develop an action plan. Those involved in the work can best set priorities and assess the feasibility of our recommendations for the specific situation at the agency. While these recommendations focus on the areas covered in our evaluation, we note that they only address some of the elements necessary for a comprehensive infection control program.

Recommendations for Management

1. Develop and maintain a written respiratory protection program for all agency workplaces to protect employees against airborne infectious agents and other respiratory hazards. Clearly define which employees are covered under the respiratory protection program and which employees should wear respirators and the circumstances under which respirators should be worn. Include all areas listed in the OSHA Respiratory Protection standard [29 CFR 1910.134] in the program, especially cleaning, disinfecting, storing, inspecting, repairing, and discarding respirators; and evaluating the effectiveness of the program.

2. Clarify the roles and responsibilities of the designated local safety officers within the respiratory protection program.

3. Offer a larger selection of N95 filtering facepiece respirators during the fit-testing campaign to correctly fit employees. For example, elastomeric respirators may an appropriate alternative to N95 filtering facepiece respirators. Also, loose-fitting PAPRs may be considered for employees with facial hair.

4. When respirator use is required, continue to require and arrange medical clearance as defined in the OSHA Respiratory Protection standard [29 CFR 1910.134] prior to fit testing. A written recommendation of whether or not the employee is medically able to use the respirator and any limitations on respirator use should be provided to the appropriate supervisors and the program administrator. It also might be helpful for agencywide records to be kept in a central location. Confidential medical information should not be shared with employee supervisors, the program administrator, or management.

5. Require and arrange annual respirator training as defined in the OSHA Respiratory Protection standard [29 CFR 1910.134]. Improve training to include specific indications for respirator use especially when employees come into contact with persons with active tuberculosis. Consider offering a training session separate from the fit-testing procedures.

6. Require and arrange fit testing annually, or when a different respirator facepiece (size, style, model, or make) is used, or when a change in an employee's physical condition occurs that could affect respirator fit [29 CFR 1910.134]. Schedule additional sessions to accommodate employees who are unable to attend scheduled dates and times because of leave or job assignments.

7. Provide a mirror during fit-testing procedures to assist the subject in evaluating the fit and positioning of the respirator [29 CFR 1910.134].

8. Develop and maintain clear written procedures for the use of respirators. Inform employees of these procedures. Define when voluntary use of respirators is permitted. Follow the OSHA Respiratory Protection standard [29 CFR 1910.134] regarding voluntary use including providing Appendix D of the OSHA respiratory protection standard [29 CFR 1910.134] to employees.

9. Conduct annual evaluations of the workplace to ensure that the written respiratory protection program is properly implemented, and consult employees to ensure that they are using the respirators properly [29 CFR 1910.134].

10. Improve training provided to fit testers to include information regarding filtering efficiency and the technical capabilities of respirators.

11. Define which employees are at risk for exposure to tuberculosis. Inform these employees that routine tuberculosis screening is recommended and that this screening should occur at least annually. Make employees aware that FOH offers tuberculosis screening at no cost to the employee.

12. Recommend the influenza vaccine to all employees annually. Make employees aware that FOH offers influenza vaccination at no cost to the employee. Explore the feasibility of offering the influenza vaccination to employees at the workplace.

Recommendations for Fit Testers

1. Verify medical clearance of subjects prior to performing a fit test.

2. Deny a fit test to those subjects with facial hair that comes between the sealing surface of the respirator and the face [29 CFR 1910.134].

3. During the fit test, include specific instructions on proper donning and doffing of the respirator, following manufacturer instructions. If the test subject is not familiar with using a particular respirator, direct the test subject to don the mask several times and to adjust the straps each time to become adept at setting proper tension on the strap [29 CFR 1910.134].

4. Instruct fit test subjects on the appropriate way to perform a face seal check and ensure that these instructions conform to those of the respirator manufacturer.

Recommendations for Employees

1. Get fit tested if you are required to wear a respirator.

2. Follow workplace guidelines on use of respirators including the corresponding guidelines on facial hair.

3. Review manufacturer instructions for donning and doffing a respirator.

4. Perform a face seal check prior to each use of a respirator.

5. Report any change in medical status that may affect your ability to safely wear respiratory protection to your supervisor.

6. Undergo annual screening for tuberculosis.

7. Get the seasonal influenza vaccine every year.

REFERENCES

3M [2001]. 8511/8211/07185 Respirator N95 Particulate User Instructions. [http://multimedia.3m.com/mws/mediawebserver?66666UuZjcFSLXTtlXfanxMEEVuQEcuZgVs6EVs6E666666~]. Date accessed: March 2011.

Beck-Sagué C, Dooley SW, Hutton MD, Otten J, Breeden A, Crawford JT, Pitchenik AE, Woodley C, Cauthen G, Jarvis WR [1992]. Hospital outbreak of multidrug-resistant Mycobacterium tuberculosis infections. Factors in transmission to staff and HIV-infected patients. JAMA 268(10):1280–1286.

Blachere FM, Lindsley WG, Pearce TA, Anderson SE, Fisher M, Khakoo R, Meade BJ, Lander O, Davis S, Thewlis RE, Celik I, Chen BT, Beezhold DH [2009]. Measurement of airborne influenza virus in a hospital emergency department. Clin Infect Dis 48(15):438–440.

Bloch AB, Orenstein WA, Ewing WM, Spain WH, Mallison GF, Herrmann KL, Hinman AR [1985]. Measles outbreak in a pediatric practice: airborne transmission in an office setting. Pediatrics 75(4):676–83.

BLS, NIOSH [2003]. Respirator usage in private sector firms, 2001. U.S. Department of Labor, Bureau of Labor Statistics/U.S. Department of Health and Human Services, Centers for Disease Control and Prevention, National Institute for Occupational Safety and Health. [http://www.cdc.gov/niosh/docs/respsurv/]. Date accessed: March 2011.

Bridges CB, Kuehnert MJ, Hall CB [2003]. Transmission of influenza: implications for control in health care settings. Clin Infect Dis 37(8):1094–1101.

CDC [2005]. Guidelines for preventing the transmission of Mycobacterium tuberculosis in health-care settings, 2005. MMWR Recomm Rep 54(17):1–141.

CDC [2006]. Prevention and control of tuberculosis in correctional and detention facilities: recommendations from CDC. MMWR 55(RR-9):1–48.

REFERENCES
(CONTINUED)

CDC [2009]. Interim recommendations for facemask and respirator use to reduce 2009 influenza A (H1N1) virus transmission. [http://www.cdc.gov/h1n1flu/masks.htm]. Date accessed: March 2011.

CDC [2010a]. Interim guidance for the use of masks to control influenza transmission. [http://www.cdc.gov/flu/professionals/infectioncontrol/maskguidance.htm]. Date accessed: March 2011.

CDC [2010b]. Prevention strategies for seasonal influenza in healthcare settings. [http://www.cdc.gov/flu/professionals/infectioncontrol/healthcaresettings.htm]. Date accessed: March 2011.

CFR. Code of Federal Regulations. Washington, DC: U.S. Government Printing Office, Office of the Federal Register.

Cook C, Heath F, Thompson RL [2000]. A meta-analysis of response rates in Web- or Internet-based surveys. Educ Psychol Meas 60(6):821–836.

Haley CE, McDonald RC, Rossi L, Jones WD, Jr., Haley RW, Luby JP [1989]. Tuberculosis epidemic among hospital personnel. Infect Control Hosp Epidemiol 10(5):204–210.

Jones R, Pitt N [1999]. Health surveys in the workplace: comparison of postal, email, and World Wide Web methods. Occup Med 49(8):556–558.

Kaplowitz MD, Hadlock TD, Levine R [2004]. A comparison of web and mail survey response rates. Public Opin Q 68(1):94–101.

LeClair JM, Zaia JA, Levin MJ, Congdon RG, Goldmann DA [1980]. Airborne transmission of chickenpox in a hospital. N Engl J Med 302(8):450–3.

Lindsley WG, Blachere FM, Davis KA, Pearce TA, Fisher MA, Khakoo R, Davis SM, Rogers ME, Thewlis RE, Posada JA, Redrow JB, Celik IB, Chen BT, Beezhold DH [2010a]. Distribution of airborne influenza virus and respiratory syncytial virus in an urgent care medical clinic. Clin Infect Dis 50(5):693–698.

Lindsley WG, Blachere FM, Thewlis RE, Vishnu A, Davis KA, Cao G, Palmer JE, Clark KE, Fisher MA, Khakoo R, Beezhold DH [2010b]. Measurements of airborne influenza virus in aerosol particles from human coughs. PLoS One 5(11):e15100.

Manfreda KL, Vehovar V [2002]. Survey design features influencing response rates in Web surveys. University of Copenhagen, Denmark: The International Conference on Improving Surveys. [http://www.websm.org/uploadi/editor/Lozar_Vehovar_2001_Survey_design.pdf]. Date accessed: March 2011.

OSHA [2010]. Respiratory Protection. [http://www.osha.gov/SLTC/respiratoryprotection/index.html]. Date accessed: March 2011.

Pappas GP, Takaro TK, Stover B, Beaudet N, Salazar M, Calcagni J, Shoop D, Barnhart S [1999]. Medical clearance for respirator use: sensitivity and specificity of a questionnaire. Am J Ind Med 35(4):395–400.

Riley RL, Mills CC, Nyka W, Weinstock N, Storey PB, Sultan LU, Riley MC, Wells WF [1959]. Aerial dissemination of pulmonary tuberculosis. A two-year study of contagion in a tuberculosis ward. Am J Hyg 70:185–196.

Sheehan K [2001]. E-mail survey response rates: a review. J Comput Mediat Commun 16(2). [http://jcmc.indiana.edu/vol6/issue2/sheehan.html]. Date accessed: March 2011.

Shih T-H , Fan X [2008]. Comparing response rates from Web and mail surveys: a meta-analysis. Field Methods 20(3):249–271.

Tuberculosis

Tuberculosis, a disease caused by the bacteria *Mycobacterium tuberculosis*, is spread from person to person through the air. Tuberculosis usually infects the lungs, but it can also infect other body parts such as the brain, kidneys, or spine. The symptoms of active tuberculosis disease in any body part include feeling sick or weak, weight loss, fever, and night sweats. The symptoms of tuberculosis disease of the lungs also include coughing, chest pain, and coughing up blood.

Tuberculosis bacteria are released into the air when a person with tuberculosis disease of the lungs or throat coughs, sneezes, or speaks. These bacteria can stay in the air for several hours, depending on the environment. Persons who breathe in the air containing these tuberculosis bacteria can become infected; this is called latent tuberculosis infection.

Persons with latent tuberculosis infection have tuberculosis bacteria in their bodies, but they are not ill because the bacteria are not active. These persons do not have symptoms of tuberculosis disease, and they cannot spread the germs to others. They may develop tuberculosis disease in the future but can be treated to prevent this from happening. Persons with tuberculosis disease are sick from active tuberculosis bacteria that are multiplying and destroying tissue in their body. They usually have symptoms of tuberculosis disease and are capable of spreading tuberculosis bacteria to others.

It is estimated that one third of the world's population has latent tuberculosis infection, and approximately 5%–10% of those infected will develop active tuberculosis disease within their lifetimes [Styblo 1980; Dye et al. 1999; Jasmer et al. 2002; Stewart et al. 2003]. More than 37 million foreign-born persons are currently living in the United States [DHS 2008]. Many of the undocumented immigrants processed by the federal immigration and customs agency annually come from countries with a high prevalence of tuberculosis.

In 2009, foreign-born persons accounted for 60% of all tuberculosis cases in the United States [CDC 2010a]. The tuberculosis case rate for foreign-born persons is more than 10 times as high as the case rate for U.S.-born persons (18.6 vs. 1.7 cases per 100,000 persons) [CDC 2010a]. In 2009, four countries accounted for more than half of the tuberculosis cases in foreign-born persons: Mexico, the Philippines, India, and Vietnam [CDC 2010a]. Among all foreign-born populations, tuberculosis rates are highest in the first 2 years after U.S. entry (75 vs. 16 cases per 100,000 persons) [Cain et al. 2008]. It has been shown that undocumented foreign-born persons had a longer duration of symptoms before medical evaluation for tuberculosis when compared to U.S.-born persons and documented foreign-born persons [Achkar et al. 2008]. The tuberculosis case rate among people in the custody of the federal immigrations and customs agency was found to be 12.5 per 100,000 persons in 2005, with patients from Mexico, Honduras, Guatemala, and El Salvador accounting for 84.4% of the cases [Schneider and Lobato 2007].

It has been shown that 20%–30% of tuberculosis patient case contacts will be found to have latent tuberculosis infection and that approximately 5% of individuals with recently acquired latent tuberculosis infection will develop active tuberculosis disease within 2 years [Iseman 2000; CDC 2005a]. These data, in conjunction with the higher rates demonstrated among foreign-born persons, suggest that individuals who come into contact with these recent entrants, including immigration officers and agents, are at risk for acquiring tuberculosis.

In 1996, OSHA issued revised enforcement guidelines concerning occupational tuberculosis exposure [OSHA 1996]. The workplaces covered in those guidelines are those where the CDC has identified workers as having an elevated incidence of tuberculosis infection. These include healthcare settings, correctional institutions, homeless shelters, drug treatment centers, and long-term care facilities for the elderly. At these facilities, the OSHA guidelines require a protocol for the early identification of individuals with active tuberculosis; skin-test surveillance for employees; medical evaluation and management of employees with positive skin tests or symptoms of active tuberculosis; placement of individuals with confirmed or suspected tuberculosis in isolation rooms; performing high risk procedures in areas with negative pressure and appropriate exhausts; and training and information for employees about tuberculosis transmission, signs and symptoms of disease, medical surveillance and follow-up therapy, and proper use of controls [OSHA 1996].

The OSHA guidelines are based on the 1994 CDC guidelines for preventing tuberculosis transmission in healthcare facilities, which were subsequently updated in 2005 [CDC 2005b]. This document discusses, in detail, the importance of administrative and engineering controls, PPE, early identification and screening, risk assessment, a written tuberculosis control program, skin testing programs, and employee education. The 2006 CDC guidelines for preventing tuberculosis transmission in correctional and detention facilities also recommend a comprehensive program consisting of administrative, environmental, and personal respiratory protection controls [CDC 2006].

Environmental controls should be implemented when the risk for tuberculosis transmission persists despite efforts to screen and treat inmates/detainees. Environmental controls are used to remove or inactivate Mycobacterium tuberculosis in areas in which the organism could be transmitted. Additional information on the types of environmental controls used in correctional and detention facilities can be found in the 2006 CDC guidelines [CDC 2006]. This document provides ventilation design considerations and air exhaust/cleaning methods for airborne infection isolation rooms and local and general exhaust ventilation systems in areas intended to contain persons with diagnosed or undiagnosed infectious tuberculosis. Individuals known or suspected of having tuberculosis disease should be placed in an airborne infection isolation room or cell [CDC 2005b; CDC 2006]. Facilities without an on-site airborne infection isolation room should have a written plan for referring detainees with suspected or confirmed tuberculosis to a facility that is equipped to isolate, evaluate, and treat tuberculosis patients [CDC 2006].

One important administrative component of tuberculosis control in correctional and detention facilities involves routinely screening employees and inmates/detainees for latent tuberculosis infection, using the TST or an interferon-gamma release assay, and administering isoniazid treatment to those individuals testing positive. Two-step TST testing is necessary for those employees who have not undergone a TST in more than a year to account for the boosting effect [ATS and CDC 2000, ATS et al. 2000]. The agency tuberculosis exposure control plan states that TST testing should be conducted at least annually on employees "at risk of exposure to tuberculosis." Upon admission to the agency's custody, detainees are expected to be screened for tuberculosis disease in accordance with agency detention standards. Suspected tuberculosis patients are further evaluated and started or continued on treatment for tuberculosis disease if medically indicated.

Respiratory protection is used when administrative and environmental controls alone have not reduced the risk for infection with Mycobacterium tuberculosis to an acceptable level. For example, protection is warranted for inmates and facility staff when they enter airborne infection isolation rooms or transport infectious inmates. Respirators should be selected from those approved by CDC/NIOSH under the provisions outlined in 60 Fed. Reg. 30355 (1995) [CFR, 2010]. Decisions regarding which respirator is appropriate for a particular situation and setting should be made on the basis of a risk assessment of the likelihood for tuberculosis transmission. For correctional and detention facilities, a NIOSH-approved N95 air-purifying respirator will provide adequate respiratory protection in most situations that require the use of respirators [CDC 2006].

Influenza

Influenza, commonly known as the flu, is a contagious respiratory illness caused by influenza viruses. Influenza viruses are thought to be spread mainly by droplets made when people with influenza cough, sneeze, or talk. Less often, a person might also get influenza by touching a surface or object that has influenza virus on it and then touching their own mouth, eyes, or nose [Wright and Webster 2001]. Evidence for airborne transmission of influenza also exists [Bridges et al. 2003; Blachere et al. 2009; Lindsley et al. 2010a,b].

Influenza can cause mild to severe illness and at times can lead to death. Symptoms of influenza include fever, chills, cough, sore throat, runny or stuffy nose, muscle or body aches, headaches, and fatigue, vomiting, and diarrhea [Nicholson 1992]. Complications of influenza include bacterial pneumonia, ear infections, sinus infections, dehydration, and worsening of chronic medical conditions [CDC 2010c]. Individuals at higher risk for developing influenza-related complications include children younger than 5 years old (especially children younger than 2 years old), adults 65 years of age and older, pregnant women, and people with chronic medical conditions (including asthma, chronic lung disease, neurological conditions, heart disease, blood, endocrine, kidney, liver, and metabolic disorders, weakened immune system due to HIV, cancer, or medication, morbid obesity) [CDC 2010c]. An annual average of approximately 36,000 deaths and 226,000 hospitalizations has been associated with influenza epidemics [Thompson et al. 2003; Thompson et al. 2004].

The 2009 pandemic influenza A (H1N1) (pH1N1) virus, also referred to as "swine flu," was first detected in humans in the United States in April 2009. On June 11, 2009, the World Health Organization signaled that a pandemic of pH1N1 was underway. CDC estimated that, between April 2009 and April 2010, 43–89 million cases of pH1N1, 195,000–403,000 pH1N1-related hospitalizations, and 8,870–18,300 pH1N1-related deaths occurred [CDC 2010e].

Spread of the pH1N1 virus is thought to occur in the same way that seasonal influenza spreads [CDC 2009a]. The symptoms of pH1N1 infection include fever, cough, sore throat, runny or stuffy nose, body aches, headache, chills, and fatigue. Some patients have vomiting and diarrhea, while some patients have respiratory symptoms without a fever. Illness with the pH1N1 virus has ranged from mild to severe. While most people who have been sick have recovered without needing medical treatment, hospitalizations and deaths from infection with this virus have occurred. Many people who have been hospitalized with this pH1N1 virus have had one or more medical conditions previously recognized as placing people at "high risk" of serious seasonal influenza-related complications, including pregnancy, diabetes, heart disease, asthma, and kidney disease [CDC 2009a]. In contrast to seasonal influenza, nearly 90% of deaths occurred among people younger than 65 years of age [CDC 2010c].

A comprehensive influenza infection control program should include all of the following: education of employees, influenza vaccination, hand hygiene, respiratory hygiene and cough etiquette, procedures for the screening and management of detainees with fever and respiratory symptoms, and the exclusion of ill employees. Use of N95 respirators or facemasks was not recommended by CDC for workers in nonhealthcare occupational settings for general work activities during the pH1N1 pandemic [CDC 2009c]. CDC's "Prevention Strategies for Seasonal Influenza in Healthcare Settings" currently recommends use of facemasks (not N95 respirators) by workers for most forms of contact with persons with confirmed or suspected influenza in healthcare settings [CDC 2010d]. In addition, CDC's "Interim Guidance for the Use of Masks to Control Influenza Transmission" does not currently recommend the use of face masks or respirators for individuals in community settings who are not ill [CDC 2010b].

Measles

Measles is a highly transmissible infectious disease caused by the rubeola virus. It causes fever, cough, runny nose, and a maculopapular (red, bumpy) rash. Transmission primarily occurs from person to person via large respiratory droplets. However, airborne transmission via aerosolized droplet nuclei has been documented in closed areas for up to 2 hours after a person with measles occupied the area [Bloch et al. 1985]. Measles is highly communicable and may be transmitted from 4 days before to 4 days after rash onset.

Measles is still a common and often fatal disease in developing countries. The World Health Organization estimated that there were more than 20 million cases and 242,000 deaths from measles in 2006 [CDC 2009b]. The disease is less common in the United States since the first measles vaccine was licensed for use in 1963. Most measles cases in the United States now are imported from other countries or linked to imported cases. Most imported cases originate in Asia and Europe and occur among U.S. citizens traveling abroad and persons visiting the United States from other countries [CDC 2009b]. Measles vaccination remains the best method of prevention. The MMR vaccine for measles, mumps, and rubella is indicated for all children 12 months of age and older and susceptible adolescents and adults without documented evidence of immunity [CDC 2009b].

Chicken Pox

Varicella or chicken pox is an acute infectious disease caused by the varicella zoster virus. It is characterized by fever, malaise, and a generalized, itchy, blistering then crusting rash. Recovery from primary varicella infection usually results in lifetime immunity. Transmission occurs from person to person from infected respiratory tract secretions, inhalation of airborne droplets, or by direct contact or inhalation of aerosols from skin lesions [CDC 2009b]. Varicella is highly contagious. It can be transmitted 1 to 2 days before rash onset through the first 4 to 5 days or until lesions have formed crusts [CDC 2009b].

In the prevaccine era, varicella was endemic in the United States, and virtually all persons acquired varicella by adulthood. Since the varicella vaccine was first licensed for use in the United States in March 1995, the number of cases has significantly decreased [Seward et al. 2002].

In correctional and detention facilities, inmates with varicella should be isolated from other inmates and susceptible personnel until lesions crust. Inmates with varicella or disseminated herpes zoster should be transferred to a community hospital, if medically indicated. Otherwise, they should be housed either in the institution's airborne infection isolation room or in a single cell with a door that closes restricted. All staff or inmates entering the cell of an inmate with contagious chickenpox or disseminated herpes zoster should wear at least an N95 filtering facepiece respirator or higher. They should wear gloves when any direct contact with the inmate is anticipated [BOP 2009].

References

Achkar JM, Sherpa T, Cohen HW, Holzman RS [2008]. Differences in clinical presentation among persons with pulmonary tuberculosis: a comparison of documented and undocumented foreign-born versus U.S.-born persons. Clin Infect Dis 47(10):1277–1283.

ATS (American Thoracic Society), CDC [2000]. Targeted tuberculin testing and treatment of latent tuberculosis infection. Am J Respir Crit Care Med 161(4):S221–247.

ATS, CDC, IDSA (Infectious Diseases Society of America) [2000]. Diagnostic standards and classification of tuberculosis in adults and children. Am J Respir Crit Care Med 161(4):1376–1395.

Blachere FM, Lindsley WG, Pearce TA, Anderson SE, Fisher M, Khakoo R, Meade BJ, Lander O, Davis S, Thewlis RE, Celik I, Chen BT, Beezhold DH [2009]. Measurement of airborne influenza virus in a hospital emergency department. Clin Infect Dis 48(15):438–440.

Bloch AB, Orenstein WA, Ewing WM, Spain WH, Mallison GF, Herrmann KL, Hinman AR [1985]. Measles outbreak in a pediatric practice: airborne transmission in an office setting. Pediatrics 75(4):676–683.

Bridges CB, Kuehnert MJ, Hall CB [2003]. Transmission of influenza: implications for control in health care settings. Clin Infect Dis 37(8):1094–1101.

Federal Bureau of Prisons (BOP) [2009]. Management of varicella zoster virus infections. Federal Bureau of Prisons Clinical Practice Guideline – January 2009. [http://www.bop.gov/news/PDFs/varicella.pdf]. Date accessed: March 2011.

Cain KP, Benoit SR, Winston CA, MacKenzie WR [2008]. Tuberculosis among foreign-born persons in the United States. JAMA 300(4):405–412.

CDC [2005a]. Guidelines for the investigation of contacts of persons with infectious tuberculosis: recommendations from the National Tuberculosis Controllers Association and CDC. MMWR 54(RR-15):1–47.

CDC [2005b]. Guidelines for preventing the transmission of Mycobacterium tuberculosis in health care settings. MMWR 54(RR-17): 1–147.

CDC [2006]. Prevention and control of tuberculosis in correctional and detention facilities: recommendations from CDC. MMWR 55(RR-9):1–48.

CDC [2009a]. 2009 H1N1 flu ("Swine Flu") and you. [http://www.cdc.gov/H1N1flu/qa.htm]. Date accessed: March 2011.

CDC [2009b]. Epidemiology and prevention of vaccine-preventable diseases. Atkinson W, Wolfe S, Hamborsky J, McIntyre L, eds. 11th ed. Washington DC: Public Health Foundation.

CDC [2009c]. Interim recommendations for facemask and respirator use to reduce 2009 influenza A (H1N1) virus transmission. [http://www.cdc.gov/h1n1flu/masks.htm]. Date accessed: March 2011.

CDC [2010a]. Decrease in reported tuberculosis cases – United States, 2009. MMWR 59(RR-10):289–294.

CDC [2010b]. Interim guidance for the use of masks to control influenza transmission. [http://www.cdc.gov/flu/professionals/infectioncontrol/maskguidance.htm]. Date accessed: March 2011.

CDC [2010c]. Key facts about influenza (flu) & flu vaccine. [http://www.cdc.gov/flu/keyfacts.htm]. Date accessed: March 2011.

CDC [2010d]. Prevention strategies for seasonal influenza in healthcare settings. [http://www.cdc.gov/flu/professionals/infectioncontrol/healthcaresettings.htm]. Date accessed: March 2011.

CDC [2010e]. Updated CDC estimates of 2009 H1N1 influenza cases, hospitalizations and deaths in the United States, April 2009 – April 10, 2010 [http://www.cdc.gov/h1n1flu/estimates_2009_h1n1.htm]. Date accessed: March 2011.

CFR. Code of Federal Regulations. Washington, DC: U.S. Government Printing Office, Office of the Federal Register.

Department of Homeland Security (DHS) [2008]. Yearbook of immigration statistics: 2007. Washington, DC: U.S. Department of Homeland Security, Office of Immigration Statistics.

Dye C, Scheele S, Dolin P, Pathania V, Raviglione MC [1999]. Consensus statement. Global burden of tuberculosis: estimated incidence, prevalence, and mortality by country. WHO global surveillance and monitoring project. JAMA 282(7):677–686.

Iseman MD [2000]. A clinician's guide to tuberculosis. Baltimore, MD: Lippincott, Williams & Wilkins.

Jasmer RM, Nahid P, Hopwell PC [2002]. Clinical practice. Latent tuberculosis infection. N Engl J Med 347(23):1860–1866.

Lindsley WG, Blachere FM, Davis KA, Pearce TA, Fisher MA, Khakoo R, Davis SM, Rogers ME, Thewlis RE, Posada JA, Redrow JB, Celik IB, Chen BT, Beezhold DH [2010a]. Distribution of airborne influenza virus and respiratory syncytial virus in an urgent care medical clinic. Clin Infect Dis 50(5):693–698.

Lindsley WG, Blachere FM, Thewlis RE, Vishnu A, Davis KA, Cao G, Palmer JE, Clark KE, Fisher MA, Khakoo R, Beezhold DH [2010b]. Measurements of airborne influenza virus in aerosol particles from human coughs. PLoS One 5(11):e15100.

Nicholson KG [1992]. Clinical features of influenza. Semin Respir Infect 7(1):26–37.

OSHA [1996]. Enforcement procedures and scheduling for occupational exposure to tuberculosis. Directive number CPL 02-00-106. Occupational Safety and Health Administration. Information date: 02/09/1996.

Schneider DL, Lobato MN [2007]. Tuberculosis control among people in U.S. Immigration and Customs Enforcement custody. Am J Prev Med 3(1):9–14.

Seward JF, Watson BM, Peterson CL [2002]. Varicella disease after introduction of varicella vaccine in the United States, 1995–2000. JAMA 287(5):606–611.

Stewart GR, Robertson BD, Young DB [2003]. Tuberculosis: a problem with persistence. Nat Rev Microbiol 1(2):97–105.

Styblo K [1980]. Recent advances in epidemiological research in tuberculosis. Adv Tuberc Res 20:1–63.

Thompson WW, Shay DK, Weintraub E, Brammer L, Cox N, Anderson LJ, Fukuda K [2003]. Mortality associated with influenza and respiratory syncytial virus in the United States. JAMA 289(2):179–186.

Thompson WW, Shay DK, Weintraub E, Brammer L, Cox NJ, Fukuda K [2004]. Influenza-associated hospitalizations in the United States. JAMA 292(11):1333–1340.

Wright PF, Webster RG [2001]. Orthomyxoviruses. In: Knipe DM, Howley PM, eds. Fields virology. 4th ed. Philapdelphia, PA: Lippincott Williams & Wilkins, pp. 1534–1579.

APPENDIX B: RESPIRATORS

An estimated 5 million workers are required to wear respirators at least some of the time while performing their job in 1.3 million workplaces throughout the United States [OSHA 2010]. A respirator is a personal protective device that is worn on the face, covers at least the nose and mouth, and is designed to protect the wearer from the inhalation of hazardous airborne particles (including dust particles and infectious agents), gases, or vapors. Respirators should only be used as a "last line of defense" in the hierarchy of controls when engineering and administrative controls are not feasible or are being put in place. The overall effectiveness of respiratory protection is affected by (1) the level of respiratory protection selected (i.e , the assigned protection factor), (2) the fitting characteristics of the respirator model, (3) the care taken in donning the respirator, and (4) the effectiveness of the respiratory protection program, including fit testing and worker training.

Respirators are categorized into two principal types: air-purifying and air-supplied. Air-purifying respirators remove contaminants from the ambient air. Respirators of this type include particulate respirators, which filter out airborne particles and "gas masks," which filter out chemicals and gases. The classification of particulate respirators can be further subdivided into particulate filtering facepiece respirators, elastomeric respirators, and PAPRs.

Particulate filtering facepiece respirators are sometimes referred to as disposable respirators because the entire respirator is discarded when it becomes unsuitable for further use because of considerations of hygiene, excessive resistance, or physical damage (Figure B1). Ten classes of NIOSH-approved particulate filtering respirators are available at this time. The minimal level of filtration approved by NIOSH is 95%. The N, R, and P designations refer to the filter's oil resistance as described in Table B1.

Elastomeric respirators are sometimes referred to as reusable respirators because the facepiece is cleaned and reused, but the filter cartridges are discarded and replaced when they become unsuitable for further use. An example of a half-mask elastomeric respirator can be seen in Figure B2.

Table B1. NIOSH-approved particulate filtering facepiece respirators and their filtering efficiencies

Filter Class	Description
N95, N99, N100	Filters at least 95%, 99%, 99.97% of airborne particles. Not resistant to oil.
R95, R99, R100	Filters at least 95%, 99%, 99.97% of airborne particles. Somewhat resistant to oil.
P95, P99, P100	Filters at least 95%, 99%, 99.97% of airborne particles. Strongly resistant to oil.
HE (High Efficiency Particulate Air)	Filters at least 99.97% of airborne particles. For use on PAPRs only. PAPRs use only HE filters.

Figure B1. A preformed filtering facepiece respirator in which the facepiece is comprised of the filter material.

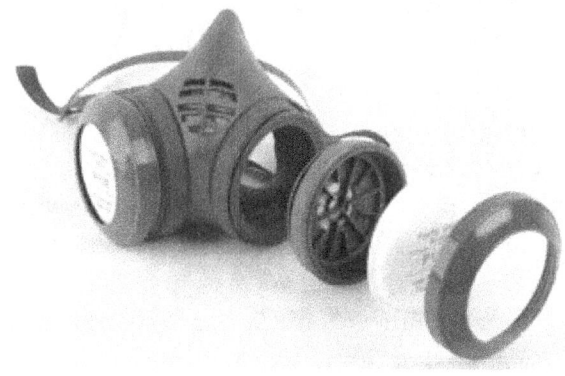

Figure B2. A half-mask elastomeric respirator comprised of a molded facepiece to which replaceable filtering cartridges are attached.

PAPRs have a battery-powered blower that moves the air flow through the filters. PAPRs can either be tight-fitting or loose-fitting. Tight-fitting facepieces form a seal with the wearer's face and must be fit tested to be sure that there is no leakage into the face mask. Loose-fitting facepieces cover all or part of the head without sealing directly onto the face. Examples of tight-fitting and loose-fitting PAPRs can be seen in Figure B3.

Air-supplied respirators provide air from a source other than the surrounding atmosphere. Air-supplied respirators are classified according to the method by which air is supplied and the way in which the air supply is regulated. These methods include SCBA, which include their own air supply, and airline respirators, which use compressed air from a remote source. A photograph of an SCBA is shown in Figure B4. Air-supplied respirators generally offer a higher level of protection than air-purifying respirators. Typically, workers exposed to high levels of contaminants, oxygen deficient or flammable atmospheres, or emergency conditions, are assigned to wear these respirators [Szeinuk et al. 2000].

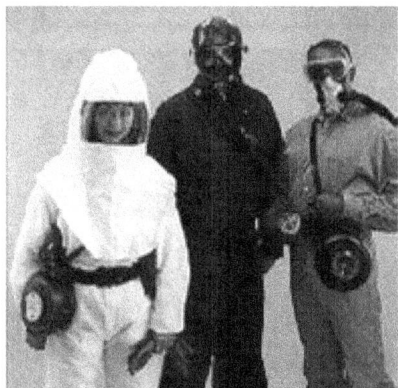

Figure B3. Various types of PAPRs. A loose-fitting PAPR is shown on the left. Two examples of tight-fitting PAPRs are shown in the middle and on the right.

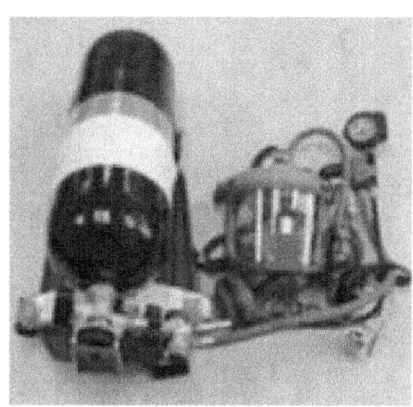

Figure B4. An SCBA containing the respirator and air supply.

NIOSH is responsible for classifying and certifying respirators for general and specific uses [NIOSH 1991]. NIOSH approval includes respirator components such as facepiece, strap, harnesses, filters, chemical cartridges, regulators, air hoses, and connectors. All respirators used to protect workers must be NIOSH-approved or otherwise accepted by OSHA. All NIOSH-approved respirators have an approval number. With few exceptions, the NIOSH approval number is not on the respirator itself, but on a separate NIOSH approval label that is found on or within the packaging. An example of this type of NIOSH label is shown in Figure B5. Figure B6 shows typical markings on approved filtering facepiece respirators. The markings shown in red are present on all NIOSH-approved filtering facepiece respirators, although they may appear either on the face, on the exhalation valve (if one exists) or on the head straps. The markings shown in black may or may not be on the respirator at all. The model or part number marked on the respirator will also appear on the approval label.

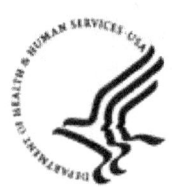
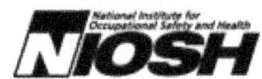

Respirator Manufacturing Company

Anytown, Anystate USA

1-800-123-4567

THIS RESPIRATOR IS APPROVED ONLY IN THE FOLLOWING CONFIGURATION:

TC-	Protection[1]	Respirator	Cautions and Limitations[2]
TC-84A-0000	N95	X 1-X2	ABCJMNOP
Additional lines may appear here showing more approval numbers and associated information.			

1. **Protection**

N95 - Particulate Filter (95% filter efficiency level)

Effective against particulate aerosols free of oil;

time use restrictions may apply

2. **Cautions and Limitations**

A - Not for use in atmospheres containing less than 19.5% oxygen.

B - Not for use in atmospheres immediately dangerous to life or health.

C - Do not exceed maximum use concentrations established by regulatory standards.

J - Failure to properly use and maintain this product could result in injury or death.

M - All approved respirators shall be selected, fitted, used, and maintained in accordance with MSHA, OSHA and other applicable regulations.

N - Never substitute, modify, add, or omit parts. Use only exact replacement parts in the configuration as specified by the manufacturer.

O - Refer to users instructions, and/or maintenance manuals for information on use and maintenance of these respirators.

P - NIOSH does not evaluate respirators for use as surgical masks.

Figure B5. Example of the NIOSH respirator approval label.

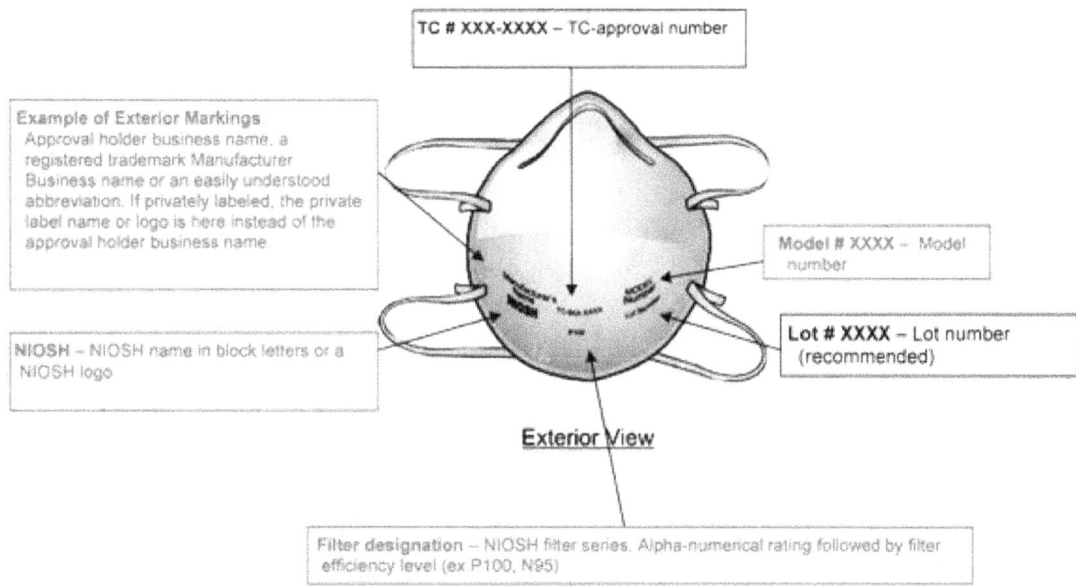

Figure B6. Example of typical markings on approved filtering facepiece respirators.

References

NIOSH [1991]. NIOSH Certified Equipment List. U.S. Department of Health Human Services, Centers for Disease Control and Prevention, National Institute for Occupational Safety and Health (Cincinnati, Ohio). Washington, DC: US Government Printing Office; 91–105.

OSHA [2010]. Respiratory Protection. [http://www.osha.gov/SLTC/respiratoryprotection/index.html]. Date accessed: March 2011.

Szeinuk J, Beckett WS, Clark N, Hailoo WL [2000]. Medical evaluations for respirator use. Am J Ind Med 37(1):142–157.

ACKNOWLEDGMENTS AND AVAILABILITY OF REPORT

The Hazard Evaluations and Technical Assistance Branch (HETAB) of the National Institute for Occupational Safety and Health (NIOSH) conducts field investigations of possible health hazards in the workplace. These investigations are conducted under the authority of Section 20(a)(6) of the Occupational Safety and Health Act of 1970, 29 U.S.C. 669(a)(6) which authorizes the Secretary of Health and Human Services, following a written request from any employer or authorized representative of employees, to determine whether any substance normally found in the place of employment has potentially toxic effects in such concentrations as used or found. HETAB also provides, upon request, technical and consultative assistance to federal, state, and local agencies; labor; industry; and other groups or individuals to control occupational health hazards and to prevent related trauma and disease.

The findings and conclusions in this report are those of the authors and do not necessarily represent the views of NIOSH. Mention of any company or product does not constitute endorsement by NIOSH. In addition, citations to websites external to NIOSH do not constitute NIOSH endorsement of the sponsoring organizations or their programs or products. Furthermore, NIOSH is not responsible for the content of these websites. All Web addresses referenced in this document were accessible as of the publication date.

This report was prepared by Marie A. de Perio, R. Todd Niemeier, Bradley S. King, and Charles A. Mueller of HETAB, Division of Surveillance, Hazard Evaluations and Field Studies. Information technology support was provided by Scott Mason. Data management support was provided by Faith Armstrong. Health communication assistance was provided by Stefanie Evans. Editorial assistance was provided by Ellen Galloway. Desktop publishing was performed by Greg W. Hartle.

Copies of this report have been sent to employee and management representatives at the federal immigration and customs agency and the Occupational Safety and Health Administration National Office. This report is not copyrighted and may be freely reproduced. The report may be viewed and printed at http://www.cdc.gov/niosh/hhe/. Copies may be purchased from the National Technical Information Service at 5825 Port Royal Road, Springfield, Virginia 22161.

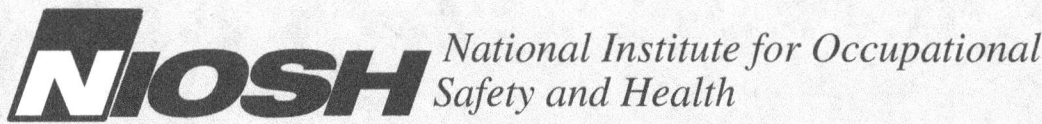 *National Institute for Occupational Safety and Health*

Delivering on the Nation's promise: Safety and health at work for all people through research and prevention.

To receive NIOSH documents or information about occupational safety and health topics, contact NIOSH at:

1-800-CDC-INFO (1-800-232-4636)

TTY: 1-888-232-6348

E-mail: cdcinfo@cdc.gov

or visit the NIOSH web site at: **www.cdc.gov/niosh.**

For a monthly update on news at NIOSH, subscribe to NIOSH eNews by visiting **www.cdc.gov/niosh/eNews.**

SAFER • HEALTHIER • PEOPLE™